LIVING WELL

WITH

LYMPHEDEMA:

A Comprehensive
Guide to Managing and Thriving

TACHA BEN-HART

TABLE OF CONTENT

INTRODUCTION TO LYMPHEDEMA

For starters, I appreciate your interest in this book and your decision to read it. I really hope the information was insightful and helpful to you.

What is Lymphedema and its causes?

Lymphedema is a chronic condition characterized by the accumulation of lymphatic fluid in the tissues, resulting in swelling, usually in the arms or legs. It occurs when the lymphatic system, which is responsible for draining excess fluid and waste products from the body, is impaired or damaged.

The causes of lymphedema can be categorized into two main types: primary and secondary lymphedema.

1. Primary Lymphedema: This type is less common and typically occurs due to developmental abnormalities or genetic mutations affecting the lymphatic system. It can manifest at birth, during puberty, or later in life.

Milroy's disease (Congenital Lymphedema): This is an inherited condition where the lymphatic vessels do not develop properly.

Meige's disease (Lymphedema Praecox): This form usually appears during puberty or early adulthood.

Late-onset Lymphedema (Lymphedema tarda): This type develops later in life, typically after the age of 35.

2. Secondary Lymphedema: This is the more common form of lymphedema and occurs as a result of damage to the lymphatic system. Various factors can lead to secondary lymphedema, including:

Surgery: Removal or damage to lymph nodes during surgical procedures, such as cancer surgeries (e.g., breast cancer, melanoma, gynecological cancer), can disrupt the normal flow of lymphatic fluid.

Radiation therapy: Radiation treatment targeting cancerous cells may inadvertently damage nearby lymph nodes or vessels, leading to lymphedema.

Cancer: Tumors can block or damage lymphatic vessels, impeding the proper drainage of lymph fluid.

Infection: Conditions like cellulitis, a bacterial skin infection, can cause inflammation and scarring of lymphatic vessels, resulting in lymphedema.

Injury or trauma: Severe injuries, burns, or trauma to the limbs may damage lymphatic vessels and cause lymphedema.

Filariasis: This parasitic infection, transmitted by mosquitoes, can obstruct lymphatic vessels and cause lymphedema (common in tropical and subtropical regions).

It's important to note that while lymphedema is not curable, it can be managed through various treatments such as compression therapy, exercise, manual lymphatic drainage, and skin care. If you suspect you have lymphedema or are experiencing symptoms, it's advisable to consult with a healthcare professional for an accurate diagnosis and appropriate management options.

Understanding the physical and emotional impact of Lymphedema.

Lymphedema can have significant physical and emotional impacts on individuals affected by the condition. Here are some aspects to consider:

Physical Impact:

Swelling: Lymphedema causes swelling in the affected body part, which can lead to discomfort, heaviness, and a feeling of tightness. This swelling can restrict movement and make it challenging to perform daily activities.

Reduced Range of Motion: The swelling and increased size of the affected limb can limit the range of motion, making it difficult to bend, stretch, or perform certain movements.

Pain and Discomfort: Lymphedema can be accompanied by pain, aching, and general discomfort in the affected area.

Infections: The compromised lymphatic system can increase the risk of recurrent infections, such as cellulitis, which can further exacerbate the symptoms and lead to additional health issues.

Emotional Impact:

Body Image and Self-Esteem: The visible swelling and changes in the appearance of the affected limb(s) can impact body image and self-esteem. Individuals with lymphedema may feel self-conscious about their appearance, leading to decreased confidence and social anxiety.

Emotional Distress: Dealing with a chronic condition like lymphedema can cause emotional distress, including feelings of frustration, sadness, anger, or depression. Coping with the physical limitations and the impact on daily life can be emotionally challenging.

Lifestyle Adjustments: Lymphedema requires ongoing management and lifestyle adjustments. This may include wearing compression garments, adhering to skin care routines, practicing regular exercises, and seeking professional assistance. These adjustments can add stress and affect one's daily routine and activities.

It is crucial to address the emotional impact of lymphedema along with the physical aspects.

Support from healthcare professionals, family, friends, and support groups can play a vital role in providing emotional support, education, and resources for coping strategies. Mental health professionals, such as counselors or therapists, can also help individuals navigate the emotional challenges associated with lymphedema.

By adopting a holistic approach that combines physical management techniques and emotional support, individuals with lymphedema can improve their quality of life and find effective ways to cope with the condition.

CHAPTER ONE

MEDICAL INSIGHTS AND TREATMENT OPTIONS

Different types and stages of lymphedema.

Lymphedema can be classified into different types and stages based on the severity and progression of the condition. Here are the commonly recognized types and stages of lymphedema:

Types of Lymphedema:

Primary Lymphedema: This type of lymphedema is caused by inherent developmental abnormalities or genetic mutations affecting the lymphatic system. Primary lymphedema can be further categorized into three subtypes:

Milroy's Disease (congenital lymphedema): This form is present at birth and is characterized by swelling in the legs.

Meige's Disease (lymphedema praecox): This type typically appears during puberty or early adulthood, resulting in swelling primarily in the lower limbs.

Late-Onset Lymphedema (lymphedema tarda): This subtype develops later in life, usually after the age of 35, and affects both men and women.

Secondary Lymphedema: This type of lymphedema occurs as a result of damage to the lymphatic system due to external factors. Common causes include surgery, radiation therapy, cancer, infection, or trauma.

Stages of Lymphedema:

Lymphedema is generally classified into four stages, often referred to as the International Society of Lymphology (ISL) staging system:

Stage 0 (Latency stage): In this stage, there are no visible signs of swelling, but the affected limb may feel heavy, achy, or uncomfortable. It may also experience a reduced ability to move lymph fluid.

Stage 1 (Spontaneously Reversible stage): Swelling becomes evident, usually with pitting edema, which means that when pressure is applied to the affected area, an indentation (pit) forms. The swelling subsides with limb elevation.

Stage 2 (Spontaneously Irreversible stage): The swelling persists and does not reduce with limb elevation. Pitting may still occur, but the skin texture begins to change, becoming thicker and firmer. The risk of infections and other complications increases.

Stage 3 (Lymphostatic Elephantiasis stage): This is the most advanced stage of lymphedema. The affected limb becomes significantly enlarged, with non-pitting edema. The skin becomes hard, fibrotic, and prone to infections, such as cellulitis. The limb may have deep folds and may be accompanied by increased functional impairment.

It's important to note that the progression and severity of lymphedema can vary among individuals, and not everyone may experience all stages. Early detection, proper management, and appropriate treatment can help slow the progression of lymphedema and improve symptoms and quality of life. If you suspect you have lymphedema or notice symptoms, it is advisable to consult with a healthcare professional for an accurate diagnosis and appropriate management plan.

Medical Diagnosis and Assessments.

The medical diagnosis and assessment of lymphedema typically involve a combination of medical history evaluation, physical examination, and diagnostic tests. Here are the primary components of the diagnostic process:

Medical History Evaluation:

The healthcare professional will inquire about your symptoms, such as swelling, pain, or discomfort, and the duration and progression of these symptoms.

They will also ask about any relevant medical conditions, surgeries, radiation therapy, or other factors that could contribute to lymphatic system impairment.

Physical Examination:

The healthcare professional will visually inspect and palpate the affected area to assess the presence and extent of swelling and changes in skin texture.

They will measure the circumference or volume of the affected limb(s) and compare them to the unaffected side for baseline comparison.

They may check for the presence of pitting edema (indentation with pressure) or non-pitting edema.

The examination will include an assessment of skin condition, such as thickening, fibrosis, discoloration, or signs of infection.

Diagnostic Tests:

Lymphoscintigraphy: This imaging test involves injecting a radioactive dye into the affected limb, which helps visualize the flow of lymphatic fluid and identifies any blockages or abnormalities in the lymphatic system.

Bioimpedance Spectroscopy (BIS): BIS is a non-invasive test that measures the resistance of tissues to an electrical current, providing information about the fluid content and tissue composition of the limb.

MRI or CT scan: These imaging techniques may be used to assess the structure of the lymphatic system and identify any anatomical abnormalities or tumors.

Blood tests: Although there is no specific blood test to diagnose lymphedema, blood tests may be conducted to rule out other conditions that may cause swelling or to assess overall health.

Additionally, the assessment may include evaluating the impact of lymphedema on your daily activities, range of motion, and quality of life. This assessment helps in developing an appropriate management plan tailored to your specific needs.

It's important to consult with a qualified healthcare professional, such as a lymphedema therapist or a specialist in vascular medicine or oncology, who has experience in diagnosing and managing lymphedema. They will conduct a comprehensive evaluation and recommend an individualized treatment plan based on your specific condition.

Conventional treatment options: compression therapy, manual lymphatic drainage, etc.

Conventional treatment options for lymphedema typically focus on reducing swelling, managing symptoms, and improving overall quality of life. Here are some commonly used treatments:

Compression Therapy:

Compression garments: These specially designed garments, such as stockings, sleeves, or bandages, apply gentle pressure to the affected limb, promoting the flow of lymphatic fluid and reducing swelling. They are typically worn during the day and should be properly fitted for effective compression.

Compression pumps: These devices use sequential compression to apply intermittent pressure to the affected limb, aiding in fluid movement and reducing swelling. They are often used in combination with compression garments.

Manual Lymphatic Drainage (MLD):

MLD is a specialized massage technique performed by trained therapists. It involves gentle, rhythmic strokes to stimulate the lymphatic system and encourage the drainage of excess fluid. MLD can help reduce swelling, improve circulation, and enhance lymphatic flow.

Exercise and Physical Therapy:

Specific exercises and physical therapy techniques can help improve lymphatic flow, increase muscle strength, and promote mobility. These exercises may include range-of-motion exercises, resistance training, aerobic activities, and specialized lymphedema exercises.

Skin Care:

Proper skin care is essential in managing lymphedema. It involves keeping the skin clean, moisturized, and protected to prevent infections and skin complications. The use of mild soaps, avoiding harsh chemicals, and practicing good hygiene are crucial aspects of skin care.

Education and Self-Management:

Education plays a vital role in lymphedema management. Individuals with lymphedema should learn about self-care techniques, such as manual lymphatic drainage, skin care, exercises, and precautions to prevent infections. They should also be aware of signs and symptoms of complications and know when to seek medical help.

Healthy Lifestyle:

Maintaining a healthy lifestyle can support overall lymphedema management. This includes maintaining a healthy weight, eating a balanced diet, staying hydrated, avoiding extreme temperatures, and practicing gentle limb elevation to reduce swelling.

It's important to note that the specific treatment plan may vary depending on the individual's needs, the severity of lymphedema, and the underlying cause.

A comprehensive approach often involves a combination of different therapies, and the treatment may need to be adjusted over time based on the individual's response and progression of the condition.

Consulting with a healthcare professional experienced in managing lymphedema, such as a lymphedema therapist, vascular specialist, or oncologist, is crucial to develop a personalized treatment plan and receive appropriate guidance and support throughout the management process.

Surgical Interventions and Emerging Treatments.

Here are some surgical interventions and emerging treatments for lymphedema:

Surgical Interventions:

Lymphaticovenous Anastomosis (LVA):

LVA is a microsurgical procedure where the surgeon connects lymphatic vessels to nearby veins, bypassing blocked or damaged lymphatic pathways. This helps improve lymphatic drainage and reduce swelling.

Vascularized Lymph Node Transfer (VLNT):

VLNT involves transplanting healthy lymph nodes, along with their blood supply, from one area of the body to the affected limb. This procedure aims to restore lymphatic function and alleviate swelling.

Lymphatic Bypass:

Lymphatic bypass surgery involves creating a bypass or diversion channel to redirect lymphatic fluid around blocked or damaged lymph nodes or vessels.

This helps improve lymphatic flow and reduce swelling.

Liposuction:

Liposuction can be used to remove excess fatty tissue in cases of lymphedema where there is significant adipose accumulation. It aims to improve the contour of the affected limb and may be combined with other surgical procedures.

Emerging Treatments:

Lymph Node Transplantation:

Research is ongoing to develop improved techniques for lymph node transplantation, including the use of minimally invasive procedures. This emerging treatment aims to restore lymphatic function and reduce swelling.

Lymphangiogenesis Therapy:

Lymphangiogenesis therapy focuses on promoting the growth of new lymphatic vessels. It involves the injection of growth factors, gene therapy, or stem cell therapy to stimulate lymphatic vessel formation and improve lymphatic drainage.

Laser Assisted Indocyanine Green Lymphangiography (LA-ICG):

LA-ICG is a diagnostic and therapeutic technique that uses laser light and a fluorescent dye called indocyanine green to visualize and map the lymphatic system. It helps identify the precise location of lymphatic blockages and guides surgical interventions.

Tissue Engineering:

Tissue engineering approaches involve creating artificial lymphatic vessels or scaffolds that promote the growth and regeneration of lymphatic tissue. This area of research aims to develop novel treatments for lymphedema.

It's important to note that while these surgical interventions and emerging treatments show promise, they may not be widely available or suitable for all individuals with lymphedema. Each treatment option has specific considerations, and eligibility depends on factors such as the individual's overall health, stage of lymphedema, and underlying cause. It's recommended to consult with a healthcare professional experienced in treating lymphedema to discuss the available options and determine the most appropriate course of treatment for your specific situation.

CHAPTER TWO

DAILY MANAGEMENT STRATEGIES

Self-care techniques: skin care, exercises, and stretching routines.

Self-care techniques play an essential role in managing lymphedema and promoting overall well-being. Here are some self-care techniques, including skin care, exercises, and stretching routines:

Skin Care:

Keep the skin clean and moisturized to prevent dryness and cracking. Use gentle, pH-balanced soaps and avoid harsh chemicals.

Protect the skin from injuries, cuts, and insect bites by wearing protective clothing, using sunscreen, and practicing proper wound care.

Moisturize the skin daily using a non-perfumed lotion or cream to maintain its elasticity and prevent excessive dryness.

Perform regular skin checks to identify any signs of infection, such as redness, warmth, swelling, or increased temperature. Promptly seek medical attention if you notice any concerning changes.

Exercise:

Engage in regular exercise to promote lymphatic circulation and maintain muscle strength. Consult with a healthcare professional or a certified lymphedema therapist to determine appropriate exercises for your condition.

Low-impact aerobic activities like walking, swimming, cycling, or using an elliptical machine can help improve overall circulation and lymphatic flow.

Resistance training using light weights or resistance bands can help strengthen muscles and promote lymphatic fluid movement.

Perform exercises that target the affected limb(s) to encourage lymphatic drainage. Range-of-motion exercises, gentle stretching, and specific lymphedema exercises can be beneficial.

Stretching Routines:

Gentle stretching exercises can help maintain and improve flexibility and joint range of motion.

Stretch the affected limb(s) and surrounding muscles regularly. Include exercises that target the neck, shoulder, arm, hand, or leg based on the area affected by lymphedema.

Work with a physical therapist or a certified lymphedema therapist to learn appropriate stretching techniques and exercises that suit your needs.

Compression Garments and Bandaging:

Follow the prescribed regimen for wearing compression garments or bandages as recommended by your healthcare professional or lymphedema therapist.

Ensure proper fitting and wear the garments consistently to provide appropriate compression and support.

Healthy Lifestyle:

Maintain a healthy weight through a balanced diet and regular physical activity, as obesity can worsen lymphedema symptoms.

Stay hydrated by drinking an adequate amount of water throughout the day to support lymphatic function.

Avoid extreme temperatures, as hot temperatures can increase swelling, and cold temperatures can cause vasoconstriction.

It's important to consult with a healthcare professional, such as a certified lymphedema therapist or a physical therapist, to develop a personalized self-care plan that suits your specific needs and limitations. They can provide guidance on appropriate exercises, stretching routines, and skin care practices tailored to your condition. Additionally, they can monitor your progress and make adjustments as necessary.

Practical tips for Managing Swelling and Discomfort.

Managing swelling and discomfort associated with lymphedema requires a combination of strategies. Here are some practical tips to help manage these symptoms:

Elevation:

Elevate the affected limb(s) above heart level whenever possible. This helps reduce swelling by promoting the flow of lymphatic fluid back towards the trunk.

Use pillows or cushions to prop up the limb(s) while sitting or lying down.

Compression:

Wear prescribed compression garments or bandages consistently as recommended by your healthcare professional or lymphedema therapist.

Ensure the compression garments fit properly and provide adequate compression to support lymphatic fluid movement and reduce swelling.

Exercise and Movement:

Engage in regular exercise and physical activity to promote lymphatic flow and circulation. Consult with a healthcare professional or lymphedema therapist to develop an appropriate exercise plan.

Avoid prolonged periods of inactivity or sitting, as this can hinder lymphatic fluid drainage. Take breaks and incorporate gentle movement throughout the day.

Skin Care:

Keep the skin clean, moisturized, and protected. Use mild soaps and avoid harsh chemicals that may irritate the skin.

Moisturize the skin regularly to prevent dryness and cracking.

Protect the skin from injuries, cuts, and infections by avoiding sharp objects and using proper wound care techniques.

Diet and Nutrition:

Maintain a balanced diet rich in fruits, vegetables, lean proteins, and whole grains.

Limit your intake of processed foods, high-sodium foods, and foods that may contribute to inflammation.

Stay hydrated by drinking an adequate amount of water throughout the day to support lymphatic function.

Avoid Extreme Temperatures:

Limit exposure to extreme heat or cold, as they can worsen swelling and discomfort. Use precautions, such as using sunscreen and protective clothing in the sun, and wearing warm clothing in cold weather.

Stress Management:

Practice stress reduction techniques, such as deep breathing exercises, meditation, or yoga, as stress can exacerbate lymphedema symptoms.

Seek Professional Assistance:

Regularly visit your healthcare professional or lymphedema therapist for ongoing monitoring, evaluation, and adjustments to your management plan.

Consult with them promptly if you experience any concerning changes or signs of infection.

Remember, it's important to follow the guidance of your healthcare professional or lymphedema therapist for personalized advice and treatment. They can provide tailored strategies and recommendations based on your specific condition and needs.

Nutrition and hydration guidelines for lymphedema management.

Nutrition and hydration play important roles in managing lymphedema by supporting overall health, minimizing inflammation, and maintaining proper fluid balance. Here are some general guidelines for nutrition and hydration in lymphedema management:

Maintain a Balanced Diet:

Consume a variety of nutrient-dense foods, including fruits, vegetables, whole grains, lean proteins, and healthy fats.

Opt for a diet rich in antioxidants, which can help reduce inflammation. Include foods such as berries, leafy greens, citrus fruits, nuts, and seeds.

Limit processed foods, sugary snacks, and beverages, as they can contribute to inflammation and weight gain.

Watch Sodium Intake:

Limit your sodium (salt) intake, as excessive sodium can contribute to fluid retention and worsen swelling.

Avoid or minimize high-sodium processed foods, fast food, canned soups, and salty snacks.

Read food labels and choose low-sodium alternatives when possible.

Stay Hydrated:

Drink an adequate amount of water throughout the day to support lymphatic function and maintain proper hydration.

Aim for at least eight glasses (64 ounces) of water per day, but individual needs may vary based on factors like activity level, climate, and overall health.

Consider Healthy Weight Management:

Maintain a healthy weight within a range recommended by your healthcare professional.

Excess body weight can contribute to increased swelling and worsen lymphedema symptoms.

Consult with a registered dietitian or healthcare professional for personalized guidance on weight management.

Include Protein in Your Diet:

Consume adequate protein to support tissue repair and maintenance.

Include lean sources of protein such as poultry, fish, beans, lentils, tofu, and low-fat dairy products.

Protein can help with wound healing and maintaining muscle strength.

Limit Alcohol Intake:

Limit alcohol consumption, as it can dehydrate the body and contribute to inflammation.

If you choose to drink alcohol, do so in moderation and ensure you stay well-hydrated.

Individual Considerations:

Everyone's nutritional needs may vary, so it's important to work with a registered dietitian who specializes in lymphedema management or consult with your healthcare professional for personalized nutrition guidance.

Remember, these are general guidelines, and individual needs may vary. It's important to work with healthcare professionals, such as registered dietitians or lymphedema therapists, who can provide personalized recommendations based on your specific condition, medical history, and dietary preferences. They can help develop a tailored nutrition and hydration plan to support your lymphedema management goals.

Stress Management and Emotional Support.

Stress management and emotional support are vital components of lymphedema management. Here are some strategies for managing stress and seeking emotional support:

Stress Reduction Techniques:

Practice relaxation techniques such as deep breathing exercises, meditation, mindfulness, or progressive muscle relaxation.

Engage in activities that help you unwind and reduce stress, such as yoga, tai chi, walking in nature, listening to calming music, or engaging in hobbies you enjoy.

Allocate time for self-care activities that promote relaxation and well-being, such as taking a warm bath, reading, practicing aromatherapy, or journaling.

Support Network:

Reach out to family, friends, or support groups to share your experiences, concerns, and emotions related to lymphedema. They can provide understanding, empathy, and a source of emotional support.

Consider joining support groups or online communities dedicated to lymphedema. Connecting with others who have similar experiences can be comforting and provide a sense of belonging.

Professional Counseling or Therapy:

Consider seeking professional counseling or therapy to address any emotional challenges, anxiety, or depression related to lymphedema.

Psychologists, therapists, or counselors can provide valuable guidance, coping strategies, and support in managing emotional well-being.

Education and Empowerment:

Educate yourself about lymphedema to gain a better understanding of the condition, its management, and available resources.

Knowledge empowers you to make informed decisions, advocate for yourself, and actively participate in your own care.

Set Realistic Goals:

Set realistic goals and expectations for yourself, taking into account the limitations and challenges posed by lymphedema.

Break larger tasks into smaller, manageable steps to avoid feeling overwhelmed.

Self-Compassion:

Practice self-compassion by being kind and understanding towards yourself. Accept that lymphedema is a chronic condition and that you are doing your best to manage it.

Treat yourself with care and engage in activities that bring you joy and relaxation.

Seek Professional Help:

If you're struggling with emotional distress, anxiety, or depression that significantly affects your daily life, consider seeking professional help from mental health professionals experienced in supporting individuals with chronic conditions.

Remember, managing the emotional aspects of lymphedema is just as important as addressing the physical symptoms. Don't hesitate to seek support from healthcare professionals, support groups, or mental health professionals who can provide guidance, resources, and emotional support tailored to your specific needs.

CHAPTER THREE

LIFESTYLE MODIFICATIONS FOR LYMPHEDEMA

Exercise and physical activity recommendations.

Exercise and physical activity are important components of lymphedema management. They can help improve lymphatic circulation, maintain muscle strength, and promote overall well-being. However, it's crucial to approach exercise with caution and consult with a healthcare professional or certified lymphedema therapist before starting or modifying any exercise routine. Here are some general recommendations:

Start Gradually:

Begin with gentle exercises and gradually increase the intensity and duration over time.

Listen to your body and be mindful of any discomfort, pain, or increased swelling. If you experience any adverse reactions, adjust or modify your exercise routine accordingly.

Aerobic Exercise:

Engage in low-impact aerobic exercises that promote circulation and lymphatic flow, such as walking, swimming, cycling, or using an elliptical machine.

Aim for at least 150 minutes of moderate-intensity aerobic exercise or 75 minutes of vigorous-intensity aerobic exercise per week, as recommended by health guidelines. However, individual capabilities and tolerances may vary.

Resistance Training:

Include resistance training exercises to maintain or improve muscle strength, which can help support lymphatic function and overall stability.

Use light weights or resistance bands and focus on exercises that target major muscle groups. Perform exercises with proper form and technique to avoid injury.

Range-of-Motion Exercises:

Perform regular range-of-motion exercises to maintain flexibility and joint mobility in the affected limb(s) and surrounding areas.

Gentle stretching exercises, such as shoulder rolls, wrist and ankle circles, and neck stretches, can help improve range of motion and prevent stiffness.

Lymphedema-Specific Exercises:

Consult with a certified lymphedema therapist or healthcare professional to learn lymphedema-specific exercises that focus on enhancing lymphatic flow and reducing swelling.

These exercises may include rhythmic pumping movements, diaphragmatic breathing, or specific limb elevation techniques.

Individualized Approach:

Work with a healthcare professional or certified lymphedema therapist to develop an exercise plan tailored to your specific condition, limitations, and goals.

They can provide guidance on exercise frequency, intensity, duration, and techniques that are safe and effective for your unique situation.

Listen to Your Body:

Pay attention to how your body responds to exercise. If you experience pain, increased swelling, or discomfort, modify or adjust your routine accordingly.

Take breaks when needed and rest if you feel fatigued.

Remember, it's essential to seek professional guidance before initiating any exercise program, especially if you have underlying health conditions or concerns related to lymphedema. They can provide personalized recommendations, monitor your progress, and make adjustments as necessary to ensure safe and effective exercise for lymphedema management.

Fashion and clothing tips to accommodate lymphedema needs.

Fashion and clothing choices can play a role in accommodating the needs of individuals with lymphedema. Here are some tips to consider when selecting clothing:

Choose Loose-Fitting Clothing:

Opt for loose-fitting garments that do not constrict or bind the affected limb(s). Tight clothing can restrict lymphatic flow and exacerbate swelling.

Look for clothing styles that provide ample room and flexibility, such as flowing tops, A-line dresses, or wide-leg pants.

Pay Attention to Fabric Choices:

Select breathable, lightweight fabrics that allow air circulation and moisture evaporation, helping to keep the skin cool and dry.

Fabrics with some stretch or give can be more comfortable for accommodating swelling.

Avoid fabrics that can cause irritation, such as rough or scratchy materials.

Consider Adjustable Clothing Options:

Look for clothing with adjustable features, such as elastic waistbands, drawstrings, or adjustable straps. These can provide flexibility and accommodate fluctuations in swelling.

Sleeve Length Considerations:

If you have arm lymphedema, consider clothing styles with three-quarter or full-length sleeves to provide coverage and modesty while also accommodating swelling.

Avoid tight sleeves or bands around the arms, as they can hinder lymphatic flow.

Layering Techniques:

Layering clothing can provide both style and functionality. Choose lightweight layers that can be easily removed or adjusted as needed.

Layering can also help conceal compression garments or bandages, providing a more aesthetically pleasing appearance.

Garments with Compression Features:

Explore clothing options that integrate compression features, such as compression sleeves, gloves, or leggings. These garments can provide both functional compression and a stylish look.

Accessible Fastenings:

Consider clothing with easy-to-reach fastenings, such as Velcro closures, snaps, or larger buttons. These can be helpful if you have limited dexterity or mobility in the affected limb(s).

Customized or Altered Clothing:

In some cases, individuals with significant swelling or unique needs may benefit from custom-made or altered clothing. Consult with a tailor or clothing professional experienced in accommodating specific body shapes and sizes.

Remember, individual preferences and needs may vary. It's important to find clothing styles and options that provide comfort, accommodate swelling, and meet your personal style preferences. Explore different brands, try on different styles, and consider seeking advice from clothing professionals experienced in fitting individuals with specific needs.

Additionally, consult with a certified lymphedema therapist or healthcare professional for personalized advice and recommendations tailored to your specific situation. They can provide additional guidance on clothing choices and strategies for managing lymphedema-related concerns.

Traveling and lymphedema: precautions and preparations.

Traveling with lymphedema requires some extra precautions and preparations to ensure comfort and minimize the risk of complications. Here are some tips to consider when planning for travel:

Consult with your Healthcare Professional:

Before traveling, consult with your healthcare professional, such as a certified lymphedema therapist or treating physician. They can provide personalized advice based on your specific condition and needs.

Plan Ahead:

Research and plan your itinerary, taking into consideration factors such as climate, activities, and access to medical facilities at your destination.

Allow for ample time between connecting flights or long journeys to avoid rushing and overexertion.

Pack Essential Supplies:

Pack all necessary supplies, including compression garments, bandages, skincare products, and any prescribed medications.

Carry extra sets of compression garments and bandages in case of unexpected delays or loss of luggage.

Use a waterproof bag or pouch to protect supplies from moisture during transit.

Wear Compression Garments:

Wear your prescribed compression garments during travel to support lymphatic flow and reduce swelling.

If you're traveling for an extended period, consider wearing compression stockings or sleeves during the journey and pack extra sets for changing if needed.

Stay Hydrated:

Maintain proper hydration by drinking enough water during your journey. Staying hydrated helps support lymphatic function and overall well-being.

Avoid Extreme Temperatures:

Protect yourself from extreme temperatures, whether hot or cold, as they can potentially exacerbate swelling or cause discomfort.

Dress appropriately for the weather and consider using cooling or warming accessories, such as cooling scarves or thermal wraps, if needed.

Practice Good Skin Care:

Maintain good skincare routines during travel. Keep the skin clean, moisturized, and protected from sunburn, insect bites, or scratches.

Use sunscreen and wear protective clothing to shield your skin from sun exposure.

Exercise and Movement:

Engage in regular exercise and movement during your journey. Stretch your legs, walk around the cabin, or perform simple exercises to promote circulation and lymphatic flow.

Follow any prescribed exercise routines or techniques recommended by your healthcare professional or lymphedema therapist.

Travel Insurance:

Consider obtaining travel insurance that covers medical emergencies, including lymphedema-related complications, to provide peace of mind during your trip.

Inform Travel Companions and Authorities:

Inform your travel companions about your condition, any necessary precautions, and how they can assist you if needed.

If traveling by air, inform the airline in advance about your medical condition and any special requirements you may have.

Know that, individual needs may vary, and it's important to follow the guidance of your healthcare professional or lymphedema therapist for personalized advice. They can provide specific recommendations based on your unique circumstances and help ensure a safe and enjoyable travel experience.

CHAPTER FOUR

NAVIGATING RELATIONSHIPS AND SUPPORT

Communicating with family and friends about lymphedema.

Communicating with family and friends about lymphedema is important to foster understanding, gain support, and create a supportive network. Here are some tips for effectively communicating about lymphedema:

Educate Yourself First:

Before discussing lymphedema with your family and friends, make sure you have a good understanding of the condition. Educate yourself about the causes, symptoms, management strategies, and potential challenges associated with lymphedema. This will help you explain the condition more effectively.

Choose the Right Time and Place:

Find an appropriate setting where you can have a calm and uninterrupted conversation. Choose a time when both you and your loved ones are relaxed and open to discussion.

Provide Clear and Accurate Information:

Explain lymphedema in simple terms, using clear and accurate information. Share the causes, symptoms, and the impact it may have on your daily life.

Offer information about the treatment and management strategies you are using to address lymphedema.

Share any necessary precautions your family and friends should be aware of, such as avoiding certain activities or being mindful of potential triggers.

Express Your Feelings and Needs:

Share your emotions, concerns, and challenges related to living with lymphedema. Express how it affects you physically and emotionally.

Clearly communicate your needs, whether it's support, understanding, or assistance with certain tasks or activities.

Answer Questions and Provide Resources:

Be open to answering questions and providing additional information to address any misconceptions or concerns. Offer reliable resources, websites, or articles where your loved ones can learn more about lymphedema.

Encourage Empathy and Support:

Let your family and friends know how their understanding and support can make a difference in your well-being. Encourage them to be empathetic, patient, and supportive throughout your lymphedema journey.

Set Boundaries and Request Respect:

Clearly communicate your boundaries and limitations, especially when it comes to physical contact or activities that may increase the risk of injury or exacerbate lymphedema symptoms.

Request respect for your needs and preferences regarding your self-care routine and management strategies.

Share Successes and Progress:

Share your progress, milestones, and successes in managing lymphedema. Celebrate small victories with your loved ones to create a positive and supportive atmosphere.

Offer Resources for Further Education:

Provide your family and friends with educational resources or recommend support groups where they can learn more about lymphedema and connect with others who may have similar experiences.

Remember, open and honest communication is key. Each person's level of understanding and support may differ, so be patient and receptive to their reactions and questions. Sharing your experiences can help build stronger relationships and create a supportive network of family and friends who are there for you throughout your lymphedema journey.

Educating employers and colleagues about your condition.

Educating your employers and colleagues about your lymphedema condition can help foster understanding, create a supportive work environment, and ensure that necessary accommodations are in place. Here are some tips for effectively communicating with employers and colleagues:

Understand Your Rights:

Familiarize yourself with the relevant laws and regulations that protect individuals with disabilities or medical conditions in the workplace, such as the Americans with Disabilities Act (ADA) in the United States.

Know your rights to reasonable accommodations, privacy, and non-discrimination.

Choose the Right Time and Place:

Request a meeting with your immediate supervisor or HR representative in a private setting to discuss your condition.

Choose a time when they are likely to be attentive and have sufficient time for a discussion.

Educate Yourself:

Be well-informed about lymphedema, including its causes, symptoms, management strategies, and any necessary accommodations you may require.

Understand how lymphedema affects your ability to perform specific job tasks and communicate this effectively.

Prepare Information:

Compile relevant information about lymphedema, such as brochures, articles, or websites, to share with your employer and colleagues.

Provide clear and concise explanations about the condition and its impact on your work.

Communicate Clearly:

Clearly explain how lymphedema affects your ability to perform certain tasks, if applicable, and discuss any specific accommodations or modifications that may be needed.

Be open about your limitations and discuss potential solutions or adjustments that could enable you to perform your job effectively.

Highlight Accommodations:

Suggest reasonable accommodations that would support your needs. This might include adjustments to your workspace, modified schedules, flexibility in break times, or changes in tasks that could aggravate your condition.

Offer Suggestions for Support:

Inform your employer and colleagues about any supportive measures that could help you manage lymphedema at work, such as access to a private area for elevation breaks or permission to wear compression garments.

Request Confidentiality:

Discuss the importance of maintaining confidentiality about your medical condition and request that this information is shared only with individuals who have a need to know, such as HR personnel or immediate supervisors.

Be Open to Questions:

Encourage your colleagues and employers to ask questions or seek clarification about lymphedema. Respond with patience and provide accurate information to dispel any misconceptions.

Follow Up:

After the initial conversation, follow up with your employer or HR representative to ensure that any agreed-upon accommodations or adjustments are implemented effectively.

Know that, each work environment is unique, and the level of understanding and support may vary. Approach the conversation with a constructive mindset, emphasizing how accommodations and support will benefit both you and the organization. Open communication can help create an inclusive and supportive work environment for managing your lymphedema effectively.

Seeking support from lymphedema communities and support groups.

Seeking support from lymphedema communities and support groups can be immensely beneficial in coping with the challenges of living with lymphedema. Here are some reasons why connecting with these communities can be helpful and how to go about finding support:

Understanding and Empathy:

Lymphedema communities and support groups consist of individuals who have firsthand experience with lymphedema. They understand the physical and emotional challenges you may face, providing a sense of empathy and validation.

Shared Knowledge and Resources:

Lymphedema communities and support groups are great sources of information and resources. Members can share their experiences, tips for managing symptoms, information about treatment options, and suggestions for healthcare professionals who specialize in lymphedema.

Emotional Support:

Connecting with others who are going through similar experiences can provide emotional support. It allows you to share your feelings, concerns, and triumphs with individuals who truly understand. It can help reduce feelings of isolation and provide a sense of belonging.

Coping Strategies and Practical Advice:

Lymphedema communities and support groups offer opportunities to learn coping strategies and practical tips for managing lymphedema. Members may share their experiences with self-care techniques, compression garments, exercises, and lifestyle adjustments.

Peer-to-Peer Support:

Engaging with others in similar situations allows for peer-to-peer support. You can exchange advice, ask questions, and learn from each other's experiences. Members may offer suggestions and guidance based on what has worked for them.

Advocacy and Empowerment:

Lymphedema communities and support groups can provide a platform for advocacy and empowerment. By connecting with others, you may gain a stronger voice in raising awareness about lymphedema and advocating for improved healthcare and resources.

Finding Lymphedema Communities and Support Groups:

Online Platforms and Forums:

Explore online platforms and forums dedicated to lymphedema. Websites, social media groups, and online forums allow you to connect with individuals worldwide who have similar experiences.

Some popular online platforms include Lymphedema Association of North America (LANA) forums, LymphCare USA support group, or various Facebook groups specifically for lymphedema support.

Local Support Groups:

Research if there are local support groups or organizations in your area that focus on lymphedema. These groups may hold regular meetings or events where you can connect with others face-to-face.

Reach out to local hospitals, healthcare facilities, or lymphedema clinics to inquire about support group options.

Healthcare Provider Referrals:

Ask your healthcare provider, certified lymphedema therapist, or treatment center if they can recommend any local or online support groups for lymphedema.

Online Lymphedema Communities:

Join online communities or forums dedicated to lymphedema. Participate in discussions, share your experiences, and seek support from members who understand the challenges of living with lymphedema.

Remember, finding the right support group or community may take some exploration. Consider joining multiple groups or communities to find the one that resonates with you the most. Participate actively, ask questions, and contribute your own experiences to foster a supportive environment.

CHAPTER FIVE

OVERCOMING CHALLENGES AND BUILDING RESILIENCE

Coping strategies for body image and self-esteem issues.

Coping with body image and self-esteem issues related to lymphedema can be challenging. However, there are strategies you can employ to help improve your body image and boost self-esteem. Here are some coping strategies to consider:

Self-Acceptance and Self-Compassion:

Embrace self-acceptance and practice self-compassion. Recognize that lymphedema is a medical condition, and it does not define your worth as a person.

Treat yourself with kindness, understanding, and patience. Focus on your strengths, accomplishments, and qualities that go beyond physical appearance.

Surround Yourself with Supportive People:

- Surround yourself with a supportive network of family, friends, and individuals who uplift and encourage you.
- Seek out individuals who value you for who you are, rather than solely focusing on physical appearance.

Educate Others:

Educate others about lymphedema, its causes, and the impact it may have on body appearance. Increased awareness can help combat misunderstandings or judgments.

Advocate for yourself and others with lymphedema, promoting understanding and acceptance.

Engage in Positive Self-Talk:

Replace negative self-talk with positive affirmations. Remind yourself of your worth, inner strengths, and qualities that go beyond physical appearance.

Challenge negative thoughts by focusing on your achievements, resilience, and the progress you've made in managing lymphedema.

Focus on Activities You Enjoy:

Engage in activities that bring you joy, fulfillment, and a sense of accomplishment. Cultivating interests and hobbies can help shift the focus away from physical appearance.

Find activities that allow you to express yourself creatively, physically, or intellectually.

Practice Mindfulness and Gratitude:

Practice mindfulness techniques, such as meditation or deep breathing exercises, to cultivate present-moment awareness and reduce self-judgment.

Foster gratitude by focusing on the positive aspects of your life, including your body's abilities and the support you receive.

Seek Professional Support:

Consider seeking professional support from therapists, counselors, or support groups that specialize in body image issues or self-esteem.

Therapeutic interventions, such as cognitive-behavioral therapy (CBT) or acceptance and commitment therapy (ACT), can help address negative body image and enhance self-esteem.

Self-Care and Self-Expression:

Engage in self-care practices that promote your overall well-being and make you feel good about yourself. This can include activities like practicing good skincare, dressing in a way that makes you feel comfortable and confident, and engaging in activities that enhance your self-expression.

Remember that improving body image and self-esteem is a journey, and it may take time. Be patient and kind to yourself as you navigate these challenges. Seek support when needed and focus on cultivating self-acceptance and nurturing your overall well-being.

Managing pain, Fatigue, and Mobility Limitations.

Managing pain, fatigue, and mobility limitations associated with lymphedema can be challenging, but there are strategies and techniques that can help. Here are some suggestions:

Pain Management:

Consult with your healthcare professional or pain specialist for guidance on managing pain associated with lymphedema.

They may recommend pain medications, topical creams, or other therapies to alleviate discomfort.

Incorporate relaxation techniques, such as deep breathing exercises, meditation, or guided imagery, to help reduce pain and promote overall well-being.

Fatigue Management:

Pace yourself and prioritize activities to conserve energy throughout the day.

Take regular breaks and rest when needed to prevent excessive fatigue.

Practice good sleep hygiene, including maintaining a consistent sleep schedule and creating a conducive sleep environment.

Gentle Exercise and Movement:

Engage in low-impact exercises or activities that are suitable for your condition and capabilities.

Gentle exercises, such as walking, swimming, or stretching, can help improve circulation, reduce fatigue, and promote mobility.

Work with a certified lymphedema therapist or physical therapist to develop an exercise plan tailored to your specific needs and limitations.

Assistive Devices and Mobility Aids:

Consider using assistive devices or mobility aids, such as canes, walkers, or compression garments, to support mobility and reduce strain on affected limbs.

These aids can provide stability, improve balance, and help conserve energy during daily activities.

Body Mechanics and Ergonomics:

Practice good body mechanics and ergonomics to reduce strain on your body and minimize discomfort.

Maintain proper posture, lift objects correctly, and use ergonomic tools or equipment when possible.

Lymphatic Drainage Techniques:

Consult with a certified lymphedema therapist to learn self-massage techniques and lymphatic drainage exercises.

These techniques can help reduce swelling, promote lymphatic flow, and provide relief from discomfort.

Temperature Management:

Extreme temperatures can exacerbate symptoms and fatigue. Stay cool in hot weather by using fans, wearing lightweight clothing, and seeking shade.

In cold weather, layer clothing to keep warm and maintain good circulation. Use heating pads or warm compresses to alleviate stiffness and discomfort.

Pacing and Rest:

Pace yourself and avoid overexertion. Break tasks into manageable segments and rest when needed.

Listen to your body's signals and adjust your activities accordingly. It's essential to find a balance between activity and rest to manage fatigue and pain effectively.

Stress Reduction and Self-Care:

Practice stress reduction techniques, such as deep breathing exercises, meditation, or engaging in activities that promote relaxation.

Engage in self-care activities that promote your physical and emotional well-being, such as taking warm baths, practicing mindfulness, or engaging in hobbies you enjoy.

Remember, it's important to work closely with your healthcare professional, certified lymphedema therapist, or a multidisciplinary team to develop a comprehensive management plan for pain, fatigue, and mobility limitations. They can provide personalized advice and interventions tailored to your specific needs and assist you in finding the most effective strategies for managing these challenges.

CHAPTER SIX

RESOURCES AND FURTHER READING

List of recommended websites, organizations, and blogs.

Here is a list of recommended websites, organizations, and blogs related to lymphedema:

Lymphatic Education & Research Network (LE&RN) - A leading organization dedicated to promoting research, education, and advocacy for lymphatic diseases. Their website provides comprehensive information, resources, and support:

Website: https://lymphaticnetwork.org/

National Lymphedema Network (NLN) - An organization committed to raising awareness and providing education about lymphedema. Their website offers resources, treatment guidelines, and a directory of lymphedema therapists:

Website: https://lymphnet.org/

Lymphedema Association of North America (LANA) - An organization that offers certification for lymphedema therapists. Their website provides information about lymphedema and a directory of certified therapists:

Website: https://www.clt-lana.org/

Lymphedema Treatment Act - A grassroots advocacy organization working towards improving insurance coverage for lymphedema treatment. Their website provides information about legislative efforts and ways to get involved:

Website: https://lymphedematreatmentact.org/

Lymphie Strong - A blog dedicated to providing education, resources, and support for individuals with lymphedema. It features personal stories, tips, and information on managing lymphedema:

Website: https://lymphiestrong.com/

The Lymphie Life - A blog sharing personal experiences and tips for living with lymphedema. It covers topics such as self-care, treatment options, and lifestyle management:

Website: https://thelymphielife.com/

StepUp-SpeakOut - A blog and resource platform founded by a physical therapist specializing in lymphedema. It provides educational content, exercise tips, and personal stories related to lymphedema:

Website: https://stepup-speakout.org/

The Lymphatic Chef - A blog focused on providing lymphedema-friendly recipes and nutrition tips. It offers guidance on incorporating a healthy diet into lymphedema management:

Website: https://thelymphaticchef.com/

Please note that while these resources are widely recognized and provide valuable information, it's always important to consult with your healthcare professional or certified lymphedema therapist for personalized advice and guidance tailored to your specific condition and needs.

Additional books and resources for expanding knowledge on lymphedema.

Here are some additional books and resources that can help expand your knowledge on lymphedema:

"Lymphedema Management: The Comprehensive Guide for Practitioners" by Joachim Zuther - This comprehensive guide provides in-depth information on the management of lymphedema, including assessment techniques, treatment strategies, and self-care tips.

"Living Well with Lymphedema" by Ann Ehrlich and Elizabeth McMahon - This book offers practical advice and insights for individuals living with lymphedema. It covers topics such as self-care, exercise, nutrition, and emotional well-being.

"Lymphedema: A Concise Compendium of Theory and Practice" by Byung-Boong Lee, Stanley G. Rockson, and John Bergan - This book provides an overview of the principles, diagnosis, and treatment approaches for lymphedema. It covers surgical techniques, imaging, and emerging therapies.

"Lymphedema and Lipedema Nutrition Guide: Foods, Vitamins, Minerals, and Supplements" by Chuck Ehrlich, Emily Iker, and Karen Louise Herbst - This guide focuses on the role of nutrition in managing lymphedema and lipedema. It provides information on dietary choices, supplements, and hydration.

"Lymphedema Management: The Comprehensive Guide for Practitioners" by Joachim Zuther - This comprehensive guide provides in-depth information on the management of lymphedema, including assessment techniques, treatment strategies, and self-care tips.

Lymphedema Resources - The website provides a collection of resources, including books, DVDs, and educational materials, related to lymphedema. It offers a wide range of topics, from self-care techniques to surgical interventions.

Website: http://lymphedemaresources.org/
Lymphatic Education & Research Network (LE&RN) Resource Library - LE&RN's website features a resource library with articles, research papers, webinars, and educational materials on lymphedema and related topics.

Website: https://lymphaticnetwork.org/resource-library/
PubMed - An online database of medical research articles, including studies on lymphedema. Searching for "lymphedema" on PubMed can

provide access to scientific literature and advancements in the field.

Website: https://pubmed.ncbi.nlm.nih.gov/
Remember, these resources are meant to complement professional advice and should not replace consultation with a certified lymphedema therapist or healthcare professional. Always consult with a qualified healthcare provider for personalized guidance and recommendations based on your specific condition and needs.